Everything You Need to Know About Social Anxiety Disorder

Are you extremely afraid of being judged by others?

Are you very self-conscious in everyday social situations?

Do you avoid meeting new people?

If you have been feeling this way for at least six months and these feelings make it hard for you to do everyday tasks—such as talking to people at work or school—you may have a social anxiety disorder.

Social anxiety disorder (also called social phobia) is a mental health condition. It is an intense, persistent fear of being watched and judged by others. This fear can affect work, school, and your other day-to-day activities. It can even make it hard to make and keep friends. But social anxiety disorder doesn't have to stop you from reaching your potential. Treatment can help you overcome your symptoms.

What is it like having social anxiety disorder?

"In school, I was always afraid of being called on, even when

I knew the answers. I didn't want people to think I was stupid or boring. My heart would pound and I would feel dizzy and sick. When I got a job, I hated to meet with my boss or talk in a meeting. I couldn't attend my best friend's wedding reception because I was afraid of having to meet new people. I tried to calm myself by drinking several glasses of wine before an event and then I started drinking every day to try to face what I had to do."

"I finally talked to my doctor because I was tired of feeling this way and I was worried that I would lose my job. I now take medicine and meet with a counselor to talk about ways to cope with my fears. I refuse to use alcohol to escape my fears and I'm on my way to feeling better."

What is social anxiety disorder?

Social anxiety disorder is a common type of anxiety disorder. A person with social anxiety disorder feels symptoms of anxiety or fear in certain or all social situations, such as meeting new people, dating, being on a job interview, answering a question in class, or having to talk to a cashier in a store. Doing everyday things in front of people—such as eating or drinking in front of others or using a public restroom—also causes anxiety or fear. The person is afraid that he or she will be humiliated, judged, and rejected.

The fear that people with social anxiety disorder

have in social situations is so strong that they feel it is beyond their ability to control. As a result, it gets in the way of going to work, attending school, or doing everyday things. People with social anxiety disorder may worry about these and other things for weeks before they happen. Sometimes, they end up staying away from places or events where they think they might have to do something that will embarrass them.

Some people with the disorder do not have anxiety in social situations but have performance anxiety instead. They feel physical symptoms of anxiety in situations such as giving a speech, playing a sports game, or dancing or playing a musical instrument on stage.

Social anxiety disorder usually starts during youth in people who are extremely shy. Social anxiety disorder is not uncommon; research suggests that about 7 percent of Americans are affected. Without treatment, social anxiety disorder can last for many years or a lifetime and prevent a person from reaching his or her full potential.

What are the signs and symptoms of social anxiety disorder?

When having to perform in front of or be around others, people with social anxiety disorder tend to:

- Blush, sweat, tremble, feel a rapid heart rate, or feel their "mind going blank"
- Feel nauseous or sick to their stomach
- Show a rigid body posture, make little eye contact, or speak with an overly soft voice
- Find it scary and difficult to be with other people, especially those they don't already know, and have a hard time talking to them even though they wish they could
- Be very self-conscious in front of other people and feel embarrassed and awkward
- Be very afraid that other people will judge them
- Stay away from places where there are other people

What causes social anxiety disorder?

Social anxiety disorder sometimes runs in families, but no one knows for sure why some family members have it while others don't. Researchers have found that several parts of the brain are involved in fear and anxiety. Some researchers think that misreading of others' behavior may play a role in causing or worsening social anxiety. For example, you may think that people are staring or frowning at you when they truly are not. Underdeveloped social skills are another possible contributor to social anxiety. For example, if you have underdeveloped social skills, you may feel discouraged after talking with people and may worry about doing it in the future. By learning more about fear and anxiety in the brain, scientists may be able to create better treatments. Researchers are also looking for ways in which stress and environmental factors may play a role.

How is social anxiety disorder treated?

First, talk to your doctor or health care professional about your symptoms. Your doctor should do an exam and ask you about your health history to make sure that an unrelated physical problem is not causing your symptoms. Your doctor may refer you to a mental health specialist, such as a psychiatrist, psychologist, clinical social worker, or counselor. The first step to effective treatment is to have a diagnosis made, usually by a mental health specialist.

Social anxiety disorder is generally treated with psychotherapy (sometimes called "talk" therapy), medication, or both. Speak with your doctor or health care provider about the best treatment for you. If your health care provider cannot provide a referral, visit the NIMH Help for Mental Illnesses web page at www.nimh.nih.gov/findhelp for resources you may find helpful.

Psychotherapy

A type of psychotherapy called cognitive behavioral therapy (CBT) is especially useful for treating social anxiety disorder. CBT teaches you different ways of thinking, behaving, and reacting to situations that help you feel less anxious and fearful. It can also help you learn and practice social skills. CBT delivered in a group format can be especially helpful.

Support Groups

Many people with social anxiety also find support groups helpful. In a group of people who all have social anxiety disorder, you can receive unbiased, honest feedback about how others in the group see you. This way, you can learn that your thoughts about judgment and rejection are not true or are distorted. You can also learn how others with social anxiety disorder approach and overcome the fear of social situations.

Medication

There are three types of medications used to help treat social anxiety disorder:

- Anti-anxiety medications
- Antidepressants
- Beta-blockers

Anti-anxiety medications are powerful and begin working right away to reduce anxious feelings; however, these medications are usually not taken for long periods of time. People can build up a tolerance if they are taken over a long period of time and may need higher and higher doses to get the same effect. Some people may even become dependent on them. To avoid these problems, doctors usually prescribe anti-anxiety medications for short periods, a practice that is especially helpful for older adults.

Antidepressants are mainly used to treat depression, but are also helpful for the symptoms of social anxiety disorder. In contrast to anti-anxiety medications, they may take several weeks to start working. Antidepressants may also cause side effects, such as headaches, nausea, or difficulty sleeping. These side effects are usually not severe for most people, especially if the dose starts off low and is increased slowly over time. Talk to your doctor about any side effects that you have.

Beta-blockers are medicines that can help block some of the physical symptoms of anxiety on the body, such as an increased heart rate, sweating, or tremors. Beta-blockers are commonly the medications of choice for the "performance anxiety" type of social anxiety.

Your doctor will work with you to find the best medication, dose, and duration of treatment. Many people with social anxiety disorder obtain the best results with a combination of medication and CBT or other psychotherapies.

Don't give up on treatment too quickly. Both psychotherapy and medication can take some time to work. A healthy lifestyle can also help combat anxiety. Make sure to get enough sleep and exercise, eat a healthy diet, and turn to family and friends who you trust for support.

Appendix A: Guide to Better Living

Note: Always consult your physician before making any changes to your diet, physical activity or life style.

Is your health condition requires that you make changes to your diet, physical activity, or life style? Are you thinking about being more active? Have you been trying to cut back on less healthy foods? Are you starting to eat better and move more but having a hard time sticking with these changes?

Old habits die hard. Changing your habits is a process that involves several stages. Sometimes it takes a while before changes become new habits. And, you may face roadblocks along the way.

Adopting new, healthier habits may protect you from serious health problems. New habits, like healthy eating and regular physical activity, may also help you manage your weight and have more energy. After a while, if you stick with these changes, they may become part of your daily routine.

The information below outlines four stages you may go through when changing your health habits or behavior. You will also find tips to help you improve your eating, physical activity habits, and overall health. The four stages of changing a health behavior are

- contemplation
- preparation
- action
- maintenance

What stage of change are you in?

Contemplation: "I'm thinking about it."

In this first stage, you are thinking about change and becoming motivated to get started.

You might be in this stage if you

- have been considering change but are not quite ready to start
- believe that your health, energy level, or overall well-being will improve if you develop new habits
- are not sure how you will overcome the roadblocks that may keep you from starting to change

Preparation: "I have made up my mind to take action."

In this next stage, you are making plans and thinking of specific ideas that will work for you.

You might be in this stage if you

- have decided that you are going to change and are ready to take action
- have set some specific goals that you would like to meet
- are getting ready to put your plan into action

Action: "I have started to make changes."

In this third stage, you are acting on your plan and making the changes you set out to achieve.

You might be in this stage if you

- have been making eating, physical activity, and other behavior changes in the last 6 months or so
- are adjusting to how it feels to eat healthier, be more active, and make other changes such as getting more sleep or reducing screen time
- have been trying to overcome things that sometimes block your success

Maintenance: "I have a new routine."

In this final stage, you have become used to your changes and have kept them up for more than 6 months.

You might be in this stage if

- your changes have become a normal part of your routine
- you have found creative ways to stick with your routine
- you have had slip-ups and setbacks but have been able to get past them and make progress

Did you find your stage of change? Read on for ideas about what you can do next.

Contemplation: Are you thinking of making changes?

Making the leap from thinking about change to taking action can be hard and may take time. Asking yourself about the pros (benefits) and cons (things that get in the way) of changing your habits may be helpful. How would life be better if you made some changes?

Think about how the benefits of healthy eating or regular physical activity might relate to your overall health. For example, suppose your blood glucose, also called blood sugar, is a bit high and you have a parent, brother, or sister who has type 2 diabetes. This means you also may develop type 2 diabetes. You may find that it is easier to be physically active and eat healthy knowing that it may help control blood glucose and protect you from a serious disease.

You may learn more about the benefits of changing your eating and physical activity habits from a health care professional. This knowledge may help you take action.

Look at the lists of pros and cons below. Find the items you believe are true for you. Think about factors that are important to you.

Healthy Eating

Pros

- have more energy
- improve my health
- lower my risk for health problems
- maintain a healthy weight
- feel proud of myself
- set an example for friends and family

Cons

- may spend more money and time on food
- may need to cook more often at home
- may need to eat less of foods I love
- may need to buy different foods
- may need to convince my family that we all have to eat healthier foods

Physical Activity

Pros	**Cons**
• improve my health	• takes too much time and energy
• reduce my risk for serious health problems	• it is too hot or cold outside
• feel better about myself	• feel self-conscious
• become stronger	• am nervous about my health
• have fun	• could hurt myself
• take time to care for myself	• am not good at being active
• meet new people and spend time with them	• do not know what to do
• have more energy	• have no one to be active with
• maintain a healthy weight	• am not young or fit enough
• become a role model for others	• keeps me from family and friends

Preparation: Have you made up your mind?

If you are in the preparation stage, you are about to take action. To get started, look at your list of pros and cons. How can you make a plan and act on it?

The chart below lists common roadblocks you may face and possible solutions to overcome roadblocks as you begin to change your habits. Think about these things as you make your plan.

Roadblock: I don't have time.

Solution: Make your new healthy habit a priority. Fit in physical activity whenever and wherever you can. Try taking the stairs or getting off the bus a stop early if it is safe to do so. Set aside one grocery shopping day a week, and make healthy meals that you can freeze and eat later when you don't have time to cook.

Roadblock: Healthy habits cost too much.

Solution: You can walk around the mall, a school track, or a local park for free. Eat healthy on a budget by buying in bulk and when items are on sale, and by choosing frozen or canned fruits and vegetables.

Roadblock: I can't make this change alone.

Solution: Recruit others to be active with you, which will help you stay motivated and safe. Consider signing up for a fun fitness class like salsa dancing. Get your family or coworkers on the healthy eating bandwagon. Plan healthy meals together with your family, or start a healthy potluck once a week at work.

Roadblock: I don't like physical activity.

Solution: Forget the old notion that being physically active means lifting weights in a gym. You can be active in many ways, including dancing, walking, or gardening. Make your own list of options that appeal to you. Explore options you never thought about, and stick with what you enjoy.

Roadblock: I don't like healthy foods.

Solution: Try making your old favorite recipes in healthier new ways. For example, you can trim fat from meats and reduce the amount of butter, sugar, and salt you cook with. Use low-fat cheeses or milk rather than whole-milk foods. Add a cup or two of broccoli, carrots, or spinach to casseroles or pasta.

Once you have made up your mind to change your habits, make a plan and set goals for taking action. Here are some ideas for making your plan:

- learn more about healthy eating (https://www.myplate.gov/)
- learn more about being active (see appendix B)
- make lists of
    - healthy foods that you like or may need to eat more of—or more often
    - foods you love that you may need to eat less often
    - things you could do to be more physically active
    - fun activities you like and could do more often, such as dancing

After making your plan, start setting goals for putting your plan into action. Start with small changes. For example, "I'm going to walk for 10 minutes, three times a week." What is the one step you can take right away?

Action: Have you started to make changes?

You are making real changes to your lifestyle, which is fantastic! To stick with your new habits

- review your plan
- look at the goals you set and how well you are meeting them
- overcome roadblocks by planning ahead for setbacks
- reward yourself for your hard work

Track your progress

- Tracking your progress helps you spot your strengths, find areas where you can improve, and stay on course. Record not only what you did, but how you felt while doing it—your feelings can play a role in making your new habits stick.
- Recording your progress may help you stay focused and catch setbacks in meeting your goals. Remember that a setback does not mean you have failed. All of us experience setbacks. The key is to get back on track as soon as you can.
- You can track your progress with online tools such as the NIH Body Weight Planner (https://www.youtube.com/watch?v=v1gluQwi eog). The NIH Body Weight Planner lets you tailor your calorie and physical activity plans to reach your personal goals within a specific time period.

Overcome roadblocks

- Remind yourself why you want to be healthier. Perhaps you want the energy to play with your nieces and nephews or to be able to carry your own grocery bags. Recall your reasons for making changes when slip-ups occur. Decide to take the first step to get back on track.

- Problem-solve to "outsmart" roadblocks. For example, plan to walk indoors, such as at a mall, on days when bad weather keeps you from walking outside.
- Ask a friend or family member for help when you need it, and always try to plan ahead. For example, if you know that you will not have time to be physically active after work, go walking with a coworker at lunch or start your day with an exercise video.

Reward yourself

- After reaching a goal or milestone, allow for a nonfood reward such as new workout gear or a new workout device. Also consider posting a message on social media to share your success with friends and family.
- Choose rewards carefully. Although you should be proud of your progress, keep in mind that a high-calorie treat or a day off from your activity routine are not the best rewards to keep you healthy.
- Pat yourself on the back. When negative thoughts creep in, remind yourself how much good you are doing for your health by moving more and eating healthier.

Maintenance: Have you created a new routine?

Make your future a healthy one. Remember that eating healthy, getting regular physical activity, and other healthy habits are lifelong behaviors, not one-time events. Always keep an eye on your efforts and seek ways to deal with the planned and unplanned changes in life.

Now that healthy eating and regular physical activity are part of your routine, keep things interesting, avoid slip-ups, and find ways to cope with what life throws at you.

Add variety and stay motivated

Mix up your routine with new physical activities and goals, physical activity buddies, foods, recipes, and rewards.

Deal with unexpected setbacks

Plan ahead to avoid setbacks. For example, find other ways to be active in case of bad weather, injury, or other issues that arise. Think of ways to eat healthy when traveling or dining out, like packing healthy snacks while on the road or sharing an entrée with a friend in a restaurant.

If you do have a setback, don't give up. Setbacks happen to everyone. Regroup and focus on meeting your goals again as soon as you can.

Challenge yourself!

Revisit your goals and think of ways to expand them. For example, if you are comfortable walking 5 days a week, consider adding strength training twice a week. If you have limited your saturated fat intake by eating less fried foods, try cutting back on added sugars, too. Small changes can lead to healthy habits worth keeping.

**When The Going Gets Tough,
Put One Foot in Front of The
Other and Just Keep Going.
Don't Give Up!**

Appendix B: How to Stay Active

Note: Always consult your physician before making any changes to your diet, physical activity or life style.

Physical activity may seem hard if you're overweight. You may get short of breath or tired quickly. Finding or affording the right clothes and equipment may be frustrating. Or, perhaps you may not feel comfortable working out in front of others.

The good news is you can overcome these challenges. Not only can you be active at any size, you can have fun and feel good at the same time.

Can anyone be active?

Research strongly shows that physical activity is safe for almost everyone. The health benefits of physical activity far outweigh the risks.

The activities discussed here are safe for most people. If you have problems moving or staying steady on your feet, or if you get out of breath easily, talk with a health care professional before you start. You also should talk with a health care professional if you are unsure of your health, have any concerns that physical activity may be unsafe for you, or have

- a chronic disease such as diabetes, high blood pressure, or heart disease
- a bone or joint problem—for example, in your back, knee, or hip—that could get worse if you change your physical activity level

Why should I be active?

Being active may help you live longer and protect you from developing serious health problems, such as type 2 diabetes, heart disease, stroke, and certain types of cancer. Regular physical activity is linked to many health benefits, such as

- lower blood pressure and blood glucose, or blood sugar
- healthy bones, muscles, and joints
- a strong heart and lungs
- better sleep at night and improved mood

The Physical Activity Guidelines for Americans define regular physical activity as at least 150 minutes a week of moderate-intensity aerobic activity, such as brisk walking. Brisk walking is a pace of 3 miles per hour or faster. A moderate-intensity activity makes you breathe harder but does not overwork or overheat you. You should also do muscle-strengthening activities at least 2 days a week.

You may reach this goal by starting with 5 minutes

of physical activity several times a day, 5 to 6 days a week. You could then gradually work up to 10 minutes per session, 3 times a day. If you do even more activity, you may gain even more health benefits.

When combined with healthy eating, regular physical activity may also help you control your weight. However, research shows that even if you can't lose weight or maintain your weight loss, you still can enjoy important health benefits from regular physical activity.

Physical activity also can be a lot of fun if you do activities you enjoy and are active with other people. Being active with others may give you a chance to meet new people or spend more time with family and friends. You also may inspire and motivate one another to get and stay active.

What do I need to know about becoming active?

Choosing physical activities that match your fitness level and health goals can help you stay motivated and keep you from getting hurt. You may feel some minor discomfort or muscle soreness when you first become active. These feelings should go away as you get used to your activity. However, if you feel sick to your stomach or have pain, you may have done too much. Go easier and then slowly build up your activity level. Some activities, such as walking or swimming, are less likely to cause injuries.

If you have been inactive, start slowly and see how you feel. Gradually increase how long and how often you are active. If you need guidance, check with a health care or certified fitness professional.

Here are some tips for staying safe during physical activity:

- Wear the proper safety gear, such as a bike helmet if you are bicycling.
- Make sure any sports equipment you use works and fits properly.
- Look for safe places to be active. For instance, walk in well-lit areas where other people are around. Be active with a friend or group.
- Stay hydrated to replace the body fluids you lose through sweating and to prevent you from getting overheated.
- If you are active outdoors, protect yourself from the sun with sunscreen and a hat or protective visor and clothing.
- Wear enough clothing to keep warm in cold or windy weather. Layers are best.

If you don't feel right, stop your activity. If you have any of the following warning signs, stop and seek help right away:

- pain, tightness, or pressure in your chest or neck, shoulder, or arm
- extreme shortness of breath
- dizziness or sickness

Check with a health care professional about what to do if you have any of these warning signs. If your activity is causing pain in your joints, feet, ankles, or legs, you also should consult a health care professional to see if you may need to change the type or amount of activity you are doing.

What kinds of activities can I do?

You don't need to be an athlete or have special skills or equipment to make physical activity part of your life. Many types of activities you do every day, such as walking your dog or going up and down steps at home or at work, may help improve your health.

Try different activities you enjoy. If you like an activity, you're more likely to stick with it. Anything that gets you moving around, even for a few minutes at a time, is a healthy start to getting fit.

Walking

Walking is free and easy to do—and you can do it

almost anywhere. Walking will help you

- burn calories
- improve your fitness
- lift your mood
- strengthen your bones and muscles

If you are concerned about safety, try walking in a shopping mall or park where it is well lit and other people are around. Many malls and parks have benches where you can take a quick break. Walking with a friend or family member is safer than walking alone and may provide the social support you need to meet your activity goals.

If you don't have time for a long walk, take several short walks instead. For example, instead of a 30-minute walk, add three 10-minute walks to your day. Shorter spurts of activity are easier to fit into a busy schedule.

Walking tips

- Wear comfortable, well-fitting walking shoes with a lot of support, and socks that absorb sweat.
- Dress for the weather if you are walking outdoors. In cold weather, wear layers of clothing you can remove if you start getting too warm. In hot weather, protect yourself against the sun and heat.

- Warm up by walking more slowly for the first few minutes. Cool down by slowing your pace.

Dancing

Dancing can be a lot of fun while it tones your muscles, strengthens your heart and lungs, and boosts your mood. You can dance at a health club, dance studio, or even at home. Just turn on some lively music and start moving. You also can dance to a video on your TV or computer.

If you have trouble standing on your feet for a long time, try dancing while sitting down. Chair dancing lets you move your arms and legs to music while taking the weight off your feet.

Bicycling

Riding a bicycle spreads your weight among your arms, back, and hips. For outdoor biking, you may want to try a mountain bike. Mountain bikes have wider tires and are sturdier than bikes with thinner tires. You can buy a larger seat to make biking more comfortable.

For indoor biking, you may want to try a recumbent bike. On this type of bike, you sit lower to the ground with your legs reaching forward to the pedals. Your body is in more of a reclining position, which may feel better than sitting straight up. The seat on a recumbent bike is also wider than the seat on a regular bike.

If you decide to buy a bike, check how much weight it can support to make sure it is safe for you.

Workout clothing tips

- Clothes made of fabrics that absorb sweat are best for working out.
- Comfortable, lightweight clothes allow you to move more easily.
- Tights or spandex shorts are the best bottoms to wear to prevent inner-thigh chafing.
- Women should wear a bra that provides extra support during physical activity.

Water workouts

Swimming and water workouts put less stress on your joints than walking, dancing, or biking. If your feet, back, or joints hurt when you stand, water activities may be best for you. If you feel self-conscious about wearing a bathing suit, you can wear shorts and a T-shirt while you swim.

Exercising in water

- Lets you be more flexible. You can move your body in water in ways you may not be able to on land.

- Reduces your risk of hurting yourself. Water provides a natural cushion, which keeps you from pounding or jarring your joints.
- Helps prevent sore muscles.
- Keeps you cool, even when you are working hard.

You don't need to know how to swim to work out in water. You can do shallow- or deep-water exercises at either end of the pool without swimming. For instance, you can do laps while holding onto a kickboard and kicking your feet. You also can walk or jog across the width of the pool while moving your arms.

For shallow-water workouts, the water level should be between your waist and chest. During deep-water workouts, most of your body is underwater. For safety and comfort, wear a foam belt or life jacket.

Tips for protecting your hair

If you're worried that pool water will damage or mess up your hair, try these tips:

- Use a swim cap to help protect your hair from pool chemicals and getting wet.
- Wear a natural hairstyle, short braids, locs, or twists, which may be easier to style after a water workout.

- Buy a shampoo to remove chlorine buildup, available at most drug stores, if your hair feels dry or damaged after a pool workout.

Strength training

Strength training involves using free weights, weightlifting machines, resistance bands, or your own body weight to make your muscles stronger. Lower-body strength training will improve your balance and prevent falls.

Strength training may help you

- build and maintain strong muscles as you get older
- continue to perform activities of daily living, such as carrying groceries or moving furniture
- keep your bones strong, which may help prevent osteoporosis and fractures

If you are just starting out, using a weightlifting machine may be safer than dumbbells. As you get fit, you may want to add free-weight exercises with dumbbells.

You do not need a weight bench or large dumbbells to do strength training at home. You can use a pair of hand weights to do bicep curls. You can also use your own body weight: for example, get up and down from a chair.

Proper form is very important when lifting weights. You may hurt yourself if you don't lift weights properly. You may want to schedule a session with a certified fitness professional to learn which exercises to do and how to do them safely. Check with your health insurer about whether your health plan covers these services.

If you decide to buy a home gym, check how much weight it can support to make sure it is safe for you.

Strength-training tips

- Aim for at least 2 days per week of strengthen-training activities.
- Try to perform each exercise 8 to 12 times. If that's too hard, the weight you are lifting is too heavy. If it's too easy, your weight is too light.
- Try to exercise all the major muscle groups. These groups include the muscles of the legs, hips, chest, back, abdomen, shoulders, and arms.
- Don't work the same muscles 2 days in a row. Your muscles need time to recover.

Mind and body exercise

Your local hospital or fitness, recreation, or community center may offer classes such as yoga, tai chi, or Pilates. You also may find some of these workouts online and can download them to a computer, smart phone, or other device. These types of activities may help you

- become stronger and more flexible
- feel more relaxed
- improve balance and posture

Your local hospital or fitness, recreation, or community center may offer classes such as yoga, tai chi, or Pilates.

These classes also can be a lot of fun and add variety to your workout routine. If some movements are hard to do or you have injuries you are concerned about, talk with the instructor about how to adapt the exercises and poses to meet your needs—or start with a beginner's class.

Daily life activities

Daily life activities, such as cleaning out the attic or washing the car, are great ways to get moving. Small changes can add more physical activity to your day and improve your health. Try these:

- Take 2- to 3-minute walking breaks at work several times a day, if possible.
- Stand, walk, or stretch in place during TV commercials.
- Take the stairs instead of the elevator or escalator whenever you can.

- Park farther from where you are going and walk the rest of the way.

Even a shopping trip can be exercise because it provides a chance to walk and carry your bags. Chores such as mowing the lawn, raking leaves, and gardening also count.

Where can I be active?

You can find many fun places to be active. Having more than one place may keep you from getting bored. Here are some options:

- Join or take a class at a local fitness, recreation, or community center.
- Enjoy the outdoors by taking a hike or going for a walk in a safe local park, neighborhood, or mall.
- Work out in the comfort of your own home with a workout video or by finding a fitness channel on your TV, tablet, or other mobile device.

Tips for choosing a fitness center

- Make sure the center has exercise equipment for people who weigh more and staff to show you how to use it.
- Ask if the center has any special classes for people just starting out, older adults, or people with mobility or health issues.

- See if you can try out the center or take a class before you join.
- Try to find a center close to work or home. The quicker and easier the center is to get to, the better your chances of using it often.
- Make sure you understand the rules for joining and ending your membership, what your membership fee covers, any related costs, and the days and hours of operation.

How can I get past my roadblocks?

You most likely will face roadblocks that keep you from meeting your physical activity goals. Think about what keeps you from being active, then try to come up with creative ways to address those roadblocks. Here are a few examples to help you get started:

Barrier: I don't have enough time.

Solution: Instead of doing one long workout session, build in three 10-minute bursts of activity during your day, such as a brisk walk. Even standing up instead of sitting at your desk has benefits.

Barrier: I just don't like exercise.

Solution: Good news! You don't have to run a marathon or go to the gym all the time to benefit from being active. To make physical activity more fun, try something you enjoy doing, such as dancing to the radio or taking a yoga class with friends. Many people find they start to like exercise better the more they do it.

Barrier: I'm worried about my health or getting hurt.

Solution: If you have a hard time being active because of your health, talk with a health care professional first. A certified fitness professional can also guide you on how to be active safely.

Barrier: I feel self-conscious working out in front of others.

Solution: Start being active at home until you feel more confident. Be active with friends who will support and encourage you.

How can I stick with my physical activity plan?

Sticking with a plan to be physically active can be a challenge. Online tools such as the NIH Body Weight Planner (https://www.youtube.com/watch?v=v1gluQwieog) can help. The NIH Body Weight Planner lets you tailor your calorie and physical activity plans to reach your personal goals within a specific time period.

You also can download fitness apps that let you enter information to track your progress using a computer or smart phone or other mobile device.

Devices you can wear, such as pedometers and fitness trackers, may help you count steps, calories, and minutes of physical activity. Trackers can help you set goals and monitor progress. You wear most of these devices on your wrist like a watch, or clipped to your clothing.

Keeping an activity journal is another good way to help you stay motivated and on track to reach your fitness goals.

Set goals. As you track your activity, try to set specific short- and long-term goals. For example, instead of "I will be more active," set a goal such as "I will take a walk after lunch at least 2 days a week." Getting started with a doable goal is a good way to form a new habit. A short-term goal may be to walk 5 to 10 minutes, 5 days a week. A long-term goal may be to do at least 150 minutes of moderate-intensity physical activity a week.

Get support. Ask a family member or friend to be active with you. Your workout buddy can help make your activities more fun and can cheer you on and help you meet your goals.

Track progress. You may not feel as though you

are making progress, but when you look back at where you started, you may be pleasantly surprised. Making regular activity part of your life is a big step. Start slowly and praise yourself for every goal you set and achieve.

Review your goals. Did you meet your goals? If not, why? Are they doable? Did you hit a roadblock trying to meet your goal? What will you do differently next week? Brainstorm some options to overcome future roadblocks. Ask a friend or family member to help support your goals.

Pick nonfood rewards. Whether your goal is to be active 15 minutes a day, to walk farther than you did last week, or simply to stay positive, recognizing your efforts is an important part of staying on track. Decide how you will reward yourself. Some ideas for rewards include getting new music to charge you up or buying new workout gear.

Be patient with yourself. Don't get discouraged if you have setbacks from time to time. If you can't achieve your goal the first time or can only stick to your goals for part of the week, remind yourself that this is all part of establishing new habits.

Look ahead. Try to focus on what you will do differently moving forward, rather than on what went wrong. Pat yourself on the back for trying.

Most importantly, don't give up. Any movement, even for a short time, is a good thing. Each activity you add to your life is another step toward a healthier you.